YOU KNOW YOU ARE

PREGNANT WHEN....

YOU KNOW YOU ARE PREGNANT WHEN....

FUNNY QUOTES FROM WOMEN

WHO HAVE BEEN THERE

KATE CASEY

ISBN: 0692372989
ISBN 13: 9780692372982
Library of Congress Control Number: 2015901487
LoveandKnuckles
Publishing, Newport Beach, CA

For Dan –

Who loves me despite my addiction to babies and reality television.

Intro

You know you're pregnant when you find yourself in the parking lot of a Mexican food restaurant inhaling fish tacos because you can't wait for the four-minute car ride home.

I know this because I spent the last four months of my third pregnancy in a Mexican food haze.

In fact, if you drove past the Baja Fresh on Pacific Coast Highway in Newport Beach that fall, you probably passed me. I was the desperate-looking woman with Tapatio sauce running down my chin.

Over the last few years, I have compiled quotes from women across the country about the strange things that happen during human reproduction.

You Know You Are Pregnant When…

- You fall asleep while sitting on the toilet.
- You stop shaving your legs for your husband and start shaving them for the OB/GYN.
- You have eaten a one-pound bag of Skittles that you keep hidden in your car from your other kids.

- You are able to carry on a casual conversation about your vacation with a person who has a good portion of his or her hand in your vagina.

Nine months can seem like eternity.

Happy gestation!

Love,
Kate

TABLE OF CONTENTS

Intro · vii
Chapter 1   Hormones · 1
Chapter 2   State of Mind · 7
Chapter 3   Strange Habits · 19
Chapter 4   Eating Habits · 27
Chapter 5   Hygiene · 39
Chapter 6   Body Changes · 49
Chapter 7   Sleep · 69
Chapter 8   Sex · 73
Chapter 9   From Husbands · 81
Acknowledgments · 89

1

HORMONES

You find yourself sobbing because of a Pampers commercial.—Christine K., Corona del Mar, CA

You are on a manhunt for the person who let their dog crap in your front yard and never picked it up.—Jane R., Crofton, MD

You wake up in a pool of your own sweat, even though the air conditioning is on high.—Denise M., Savannah, GA

You ask your husband at least three times a day if you are getting too fat.—Katherine L., Austin, TX

You consider punching your husband when he suggests you might be getting too fat.—LeeAnn P., Round Rock, TX

You cry while watching SpongeBob SquarePants.—Lizzeth V., Orange, CA

The eliminations portion of *American Idol* is beginning to put you into a mild form of depression.—Nicole B., Tucson, AZ

The sight of your husband sleeping peacefully next to you makes you want to hurt him physically.—Erin G., Newport Beach, CA

The sound of your coworker typing makes you want to throw their computer out the window.—Nicole O., Seattle, WA

You spend thirty minutes venting to the barista at the coffee shop about your in-laws.—Briana G., Round Rock, TX

You want to run down the perfectly able-bodied person who parks close to the front door of the store.—Gabrielle P., Fort Lauderdale, FL

2

State of Mind

You Know You Are Pregnant When...

You arrive at work to be pulled aside by your secretary, who tells you that your shoes don't match.—Meghan M., Alexandria, VA

You take naps in your car during work breaks.—Jessica M., Waco, TX

While in the shower, you can't seem to remember whether you have just shampooed your hair or not.—Kate C., Newport Beach, CA

You wish you had waited one more weekend to take the pregnancy test so you could have enjoyed a few more glasses (bottles) of wine.—Carrie R., Yorba Linda, CA

You smell onions, even when there are no onions around.—Kelly N., Harrisburg, PA

The smell of your spice cabinet makes you gag.—Linda H., Gambier, OH

Complete strangers approach you to revel in the joy and excitement of a new life.—Renee N., Savannah, GA

You switch Maalox for the *Fifty Shades of Grey* book on your nightstand.—Mindi H., Tarpon Springs, FL

You start checking out strollers on the street like you used to check out hot guys.—Braunwyn B., Miami, FL.

You can never remember where you left your keys, even though you always leave them in the same place.—Megan R., Sea Bright, NJ

You can't figure out why the mail didn't come, even though it is Sunday.—Lisa G., Provo, UT

You stall when asked by the customer service person on the other end of the phone line what your name is.—Grace J., New Rochelle, NY

You can't remember your social security number or the pin number for your ATM card.—Monica Z., Steeplechase, MD

You realize you have been driving around town with your gas cap hanging from your car.—Melissa L., Little Silver, NJ

Strangers tell you their birth story.—Julia K., Newport Beach, CA

You can't remember simple words like room, refrigerator, or car. – Teni K., New York, NY

Your holiday plans revolve around your scheduled C-section. – Arielle B., Pittsburgh, PA

Your single friends are embarrassed to hang out with you. – Bonnie B., New Orleans, LA

Your current form of exercise is walking from the couch to the bathroom. – Lora B., Norfolk, VA

You wonder at least two times a day if your life is over. – Theresa A., Patterson, NJ

You long for the trips you used to take to Las Vegas. – Tracy M., San Francisco, CA

You worry you will never go back to Las Vegas. – Tracy M., San Francisco, CA

3

STRANGE HABITS

YOU KNOW YOU ARE PREGNANT WHEN...

You pee when you sneeze and pee when you laugh.—Sarah B., Morgantown, WV

You sniff around the house searching for a smell no one else seems to notice.—Shannon M., Malvern, PA

Your travel plans revolve around your ability to use a restroom. – Rebecca M., Punta Gorda, FL

A casting agent from Hoarders would want to discuss your recent online baby clothes purchases. – Tina A., Akron, OH

You can no longer remember directions back to your house. – Cristina L., Miami, FL

You hit up moms at the park so you will have new friends. – Courtney N., Raleigh, NC

New Internet searches include nanny cams, security systems, and cord blood banks. – Tia S., Baltimore, MD

Just walking into the grocery store makes you run to the bathroom to puke for the eighth time that day.—Karah B., Hoboken, NJ

Previously innocuous smells (citrus cleaner, blossoming flowers, cooking meat of any kind, your husband's deodorant, your own farts) make you want to die.—Ashley M., Houston, TX

You add "pregnancy" and "normal?" to everything you Google.—Samantha S., Laguna Niguel, CA

You become obsessed with the color of your discharge.—
Melanie H., Appleton, WI

You are naked and have about ten people in the delivery room (all strangers, minus husband), and you don't even care what they're seeing on the other side of the sheet.—Shannon P., Lexington, KY

Friday night fun has gone from sushi and sake to another thrilling evening spent with your label maker. And although you are content, you are equally annoyed that your husband is bored. Does he not worry you have yet to label the produce drawer?—Stephani C., Newport Beach, CA

4

EATING HABITS

You go to Costco for a new refrigerator but leave with two pizzas.—Danielle D., Ventura, CA

You start thinking about dinner when you're finishing your lunch!—Sarah M., West Chester, PA

Eating a pound of bacon in a sitting is considered an appetizer.—Meghan M., Alexandria, VA

You make spaghetti at 8:00 a.m.—Julia M., Monrovia, CA

The drive-through crew at McDonald's has two fresh double cheeseburgers and a fountain Coke ready every day at 11:00 a.m. when breakfast ends, and they know your voice on the speaker.—Kate P., Pittsburgh, PA

You know that In-N-Out opens at 10:30 a.m.—Heather C., Newport Beach CA

Serving size is irrelevant.—Samantha S., Laguna Niguel, CA

The In-N-Out guy Bryan (with a "Y") just smiles when he sees you, probably because he can't see your belly under the steering wheel and you're there so much, he must think you have a crush on him (it doesn't help that you're not wearing your wedding ring because your fingers are sausages).—Heather C., Newport Beach, CA

That second donut at the D&D drive-through is justified because it is "for the baby."—Caitlin O., Boston, MA

Coffee smells like burnt tuna.—Claire H.,Dayton, OH.

You haven't eaten fast food in years, but suddenly you notice a KFC that you pass by every single day.—Alicia Q., Kenosha, WI

You can't even begin to pull your skinny jeans up over your now many-inches-wider thighs, but people insist on telling you that from behind, they can't even tell you're pregnant.—Maeve S., Boston, MA

You wonder if Dunkin' Donuts has a membership program.—Lily N., Bedford, NY

You tell your husband that because he will not get out of bed at midnight and go to the store to buy you your very specific order of Rusty's salt and vinegar potato chips and Entenmann's glazed donut holes, you seriously doubt that he is going to be a good father.—Christine K., Corona del Mar, CA

For the first time in your adult life, champagne and wine don't sound good at all.—Alli T., Hot Springs, AK

You consider a small pizza dessert. – Hadley I., Eau Claire, WI

The staffs at Chipotle already know your lunch order – Vanessa C., Scottsdale, AZ

You buy Girl Scout cookies on eBay. – Christina H., Newport Beach, CA

The only reason you are at Ikea is to eat the Swedish meatballs. – Helen T., Washington, DC

You send your husband to pickup takeout for dinner and he is shocked to realize you ordered $150 worth of Greek food with no intention of sharing it. – Carlene S., Newport Beach, CA

You wake up thinking about ribs and coleslaw. – Jessica T., South Carolina

5

Hygiene

You have to sit to brush your teeth for fear of passing out from exhaustion while standing.—Mary D., Des Moines, IA

You feel like you should carry cat litter in your purse to sprinkle in your underwear.—Stacy F., Vandalia, OH

You get up to pee, and you already did.—Erica M., Stow, MA

You have to take breaks while blow-drying your hair because your arms have become too heavy to lift.—Danielle B., Eureka Springs, IA

You sneeze, and you're not sure if your water just broke or you peed your pants again!—Corey C., Honolulu, HI

You burp and vomit at same time.—Laurie D., Gulfport, MI

You have antacids on the nightstand, in your purse, in the kitchen, on your desk, in your coat pocket, etc., etc., etc. You get the idea.—Deni M., Olympia, WI

Brushing your teeth makes you gag.—Jessica K., Corona del Mar, CA

You save your best outfit/undies for OB appointment day.—Natalie G., New York, NY

You sound like Marilyn Monroe during your weekly PowerPoint presentation at work because the baby is squishing your lungs.—Sally P., New York, NY

You must be no more than ten feet from a bathroom at all times.—Kerry P., Peoria, IL

You know where every bathroom is anywhere you've ever been.—Kimberly V., Montpelier, VT

You are walking down the street and can smell the perfume on people in their cars driving by.—Megan J., Middlebury, VT

You use your growing belly to your advantage at work. When someone asks you a really difficult question at your presentation, you say "Oh! Sorry, that was the baby." Instant distraction.—Aisha M., Los Angeles, CA

You haven't seen your own bush in months.—Katy R., Dallas, TX

You hug the toilet more than you hug your husband.— Samantha S., Laguna Niguel, CA

You assume everyone wants your urine sample. – Jenna W., Columbus, OH

You have nightmares about pooping during labor. – Maria P., Minneapolis, MN

You are thrilled you don't have to wear tampons for 9 months. – Melissa F., Storrs, CT

Extra cash is spent on baby books and hemorrhoid medication. – Carol F., New York, NY

6

BODY CHANGES

You are completely fine wearing flip-flops anywhere and everywhere—including client meetings and church.—Katy R., Dallas, TX

Your bikini waxer tells you that you're getting ingrown hairs on your inner thighs because they are rubbing together when you walk, and sends you home with talcum powder.—Annabelle C., Downingtown, PA

You carry extra underwear in your bag because if there is a chance you might laugh, cough, sneeze, or breathe, you are going to pee your pants.—Maura B., Hagerstown, MD

You're in the shower, look down, and can't see your vagina. Then you need to get out of said shower to look in a mirror to confirm it's still there.—Hayley D., Mercer Island, WA

You feel like there is a ten-pound dumbbell in your vagina.—Helen S., Mission Viejo, CA

You wake up, and your boobs look like a road map (from veins) and your nipples look like a blind child could find them.—Jennifer C., Downingtown, PA

You get up to pee in the middle of the night, and you're so heavy that the armoire shakes when you walk past it and wakes up your husband.—Jennifer F., Corona del Mar, CA

You have to slowly lower your boobs out of your bra because they are so tender.—Deanna D., Bangor, ME

You're so swollen in your third trimester you develop carpal tunnel in both wrists.—Megan W., Providence, RI

Suddenly those stork parking spots for expectant mothers seem like a really reasonable thing to provide to customers.—Kirsten E., Potomac, MD

You set the belt of your robe on fire making breakfast at the stove because you can't see below your belly.—Alexis M., Annapolis, MD

Complete strangers find it appropriate to comment on your weight by asking if you're having twins and completely insulting you right before you give birth to only one child.—Kindra U., Orange, CA

You start waddling down the hall.—Jaclyn V., Oyster Bay, NY

You want to physically assault the person that asked if you were having triplets.—Kelsey W., Newport Coast, CA.

You're attending a prenatal yoga class, which is code for sitting around discussing how your ankles are now cankles.—Nicole M., New Haven, CT

You need a nap to prep for bedtime.—Gwen G., Grosse Pointe, MI

What you thought was a hangover/motion sickness from the cruise to Ensenada and an entire day of tequila shots lasts more than a few days.—Christa M., Jackson Hole, ID

You power up for your treadmill workout by eating a bag of chocolate.—Dara B., Wilmington, DE

You compensate for caffeine withdrawal by eating a bag of chocolate.—Dara B., Wilmington, DE

You tell yourself you will get your prebaby body back no matter what those skinny moms tell you, and then comfort yourself with a bag of chocolate.—Dara B., Wilmington, DE

You have to hold your breath to be able to bend over and put on shoes.—Caitlin O., Boston, MA

Your shoes suddenly don't fit anymore because, apparently, your feet also grow with the rest of your body during pregnancy.—Caitlin O., Boston, MA

You know you're pregnant when you revisit your puberty years with a new case of "bacne" (back acne).—Stephani C., Newport Beach, CA

Pooping daily warrants sharing with friends and family.—Donna P., New Orleans, LA

Your jeans that you have saved for ten years as your "fat jeans" now do not fit up over your knees.—Christine K., Corona del Mar, CA

Your butt, boobs, and belly get bigger, but your bladder gets smaller.—Shannon M., Malvern, PA

You show up for a 6:00 a.m. workout with evidence of the powdered donuts you just shoveled in on your face.—Christine B., Palmyra, PA

You are planning the dessert you will devour after your three-course dinner while eating breakfast.—Stephani C., Newport Beach, CA

You have consumed an entire box of Thin Mints, and your husband knows better than to call you out.—Allison S., Miami, FL

Your dog is looking at you like he's thinking "Wow, you've let yourself go."—Raquel S., Madison, WI

You have a hard time explaining why you suddenly have more acne than your 12-year-old niece. – Denise G., Richmond, VA.

Not being able to button your old jeans makes you want to spend the rest of the year living in your closet. Leann T., Bristol, VA.

It takes a few minutes to get out of a restaurant booth. – Lisa M., West Chester, PA

It feels like your boobs are suddenly filed with lead. – Maureen C., Boulder, CO

Flip-flops are the only shoes that can accommodate your swollen feet. – Charlene S., Bedford, NY

You daydream about tummy tuck procedures. – Victoria D., Brattleboro, VT

The bottom of your purse is covered in Swedish fish and M&Ms. – Marissa P., Hoboken, NJ

You feel the need to explain to strangers that you aren't fat, just carrying a baby. – Carrie L., Newport Beach, CA

7

SLEEP

There is no point in starting a show after 8:30 p.m. because you won't make it past the first commercial.—Aubrey G., Atlanta, GA

If another person tells you to "get your sleep now," you will surely clock them in the face.—Jennifer Y., Kansas City, MO

Making it to midnight on New Year's Eve feels like a marathon with a very lame finish line.—Kerri L., Portland, OR

You have to sit down midshower or in the middle of brushing your teeth because you're so tired.—Jill D., Portsmouth, NH

You would rather sleep than have sex or eat.—Jen H., Newport Beach, CA

You request a recliner to replace your office chair.—Stephanie V., Saint Louis, MO

8

SEX

YOU KNOW YOU ARE PREGNANT WHEN...

Sex seems like putting a puzzle together where the pieces just don't fit.—Chris B., New York, NY

Laughing during sex is encouraged.—Madison W., Simsbury, CT

You struggle to stay awake and your husband doesn't care. – Nicole W., New York, NY.

Your husband has a hard time getting excited about a woman wearing her maternity pants backwards.—Shannon S., Indianapolis, IN

Your husband starts calling you "jungle tits."—Devon H.,Costa Mesa, CA.

You have sex out of duty and no other reason.—Christine K., Corona del Mar, CA

You don't want to have sex because your anatomy is so swollen.—Michelle C., Newport Beach, CA

You actually beg your husband for sex because you desperately hope it will send you into labor, and then apologize to him because you just made him have sex with a whale.—Marry Ellen M., West Chester, PA

Your body pillow is the only thing you want touching you at night. – Molly M., West Roxbury, MA.

Your idea of sex is the lights out, under the covers, and wearing a hoodie. – Kim N., Houston, TX

You hope your husband will still be attracted to you when you have to start wearing a nursing bra. – Joanne G., Scranton, PA

You long for your old boobs. – Molly M., Seattle, WA

Your husband is excited about your new boobs. – Molly M., Seattle, WA

Your new idea of a wild night is the Vanderpump Rules marathon and a bag of Doritos. – Nancy R., Los Angeles, CA.

9

FROM HUSBANDS

The Geico lizard commercials make your wife cry because "he is just so cute."—James B., San Diego, CA

You have to drive to get papayas at four o'clock in the morning, sometimes even from the back of the grocery stores as the trucks are getting loaded in.—Ricardo D., Los Angeles, CA

Her idea for dinner is hot dogs...every night.—Jacob B., Washington, DC

You don't have to wear condoms anymore.—Jason S., Hershey, PA

A conversation about toothpaste suddenly becomes a mine-field.—Brett J., Dallas, TX

Every argument is lost with the words "I'm ruining my body for you."—Michael K., New York, NY

She yells from the bathroom, "There is no line," then two minutes later she yells, "Oh wait, there is a line." We are having a baby!—Chris B., Philadelphia, PA

You're running out to Dairy Queen at 10:00 p.m. for a Blizzard, and she is devastated that you forgot your wallet.—Steve L., Baltimore, MD

Talking makes her short of breath.—Keith D., Hanover, NH

You can't recognize her vagina.—Keith D., Hanover, NH

You come home from work to find her snoring and drooling on the couch.—Jason M., Charlottesville, NC

She is constantly feeding your fear her weight could possibly climb higher than yours.—Frank M., Newport Beach, CA

After twelve hours of sleep, she wakes up and says, "I'm so tired."—Roland K., Corona del Mar, CA

She has left a permanent impression in the couch and a trail of crumbs follows her wherever she goes. – Simon K., West Roxbury, MA.

She's the one clogging the toilet. – Jeff D., Mission Viejo, CA

Her idea of a hot date is attending a birthing class. – Roger D., Orange, CA

Acknowledgments

Thank you to all the women (and husbands) who graciously offered quotes.

www.ingramcontent.com/pod-product-compliance
Lightning Source LLC
Chambersburg PA
CBHW050546280326
41933CB00011B/1734